Things I Notice When I Walk the Dog

for Agatha

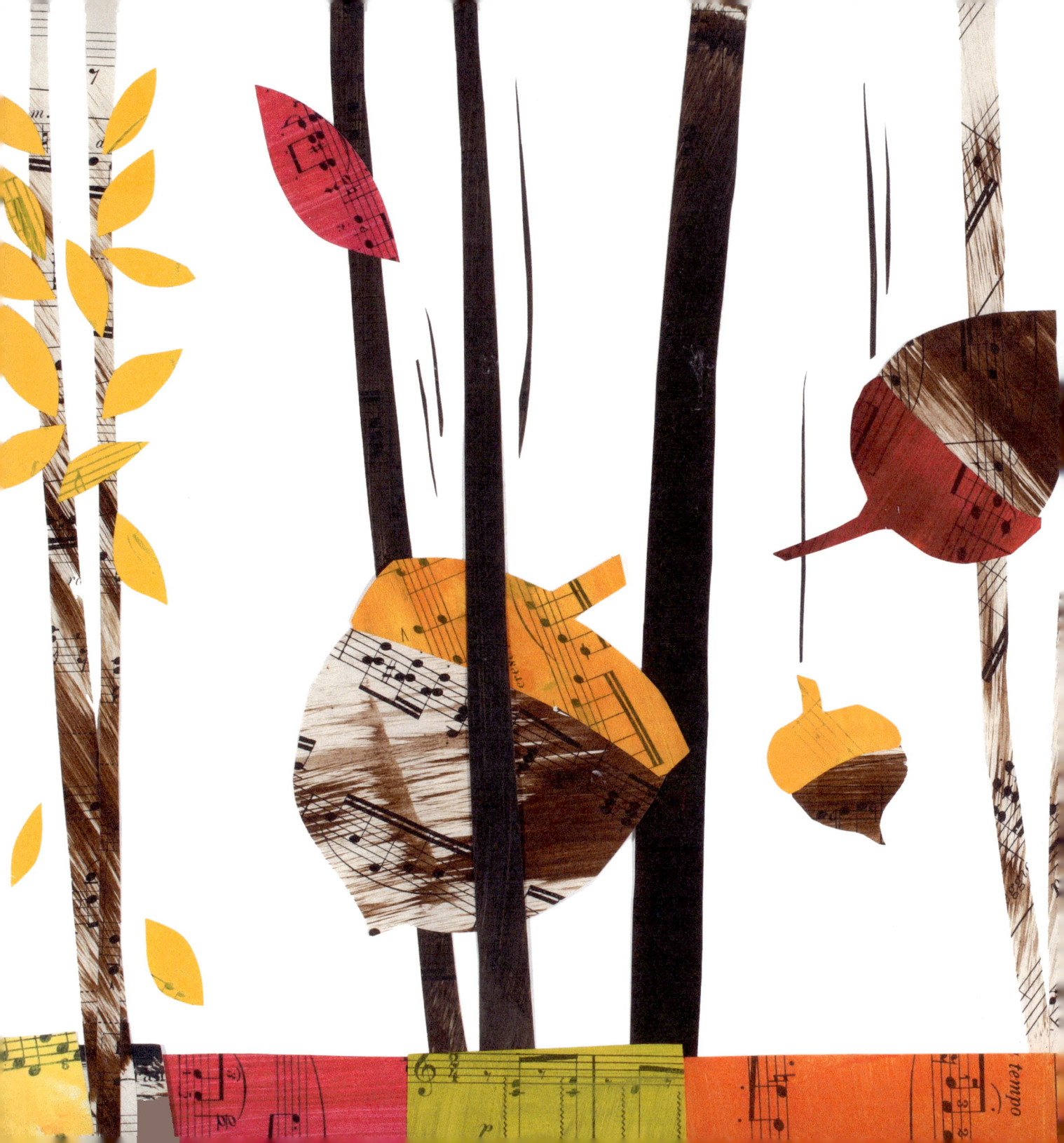

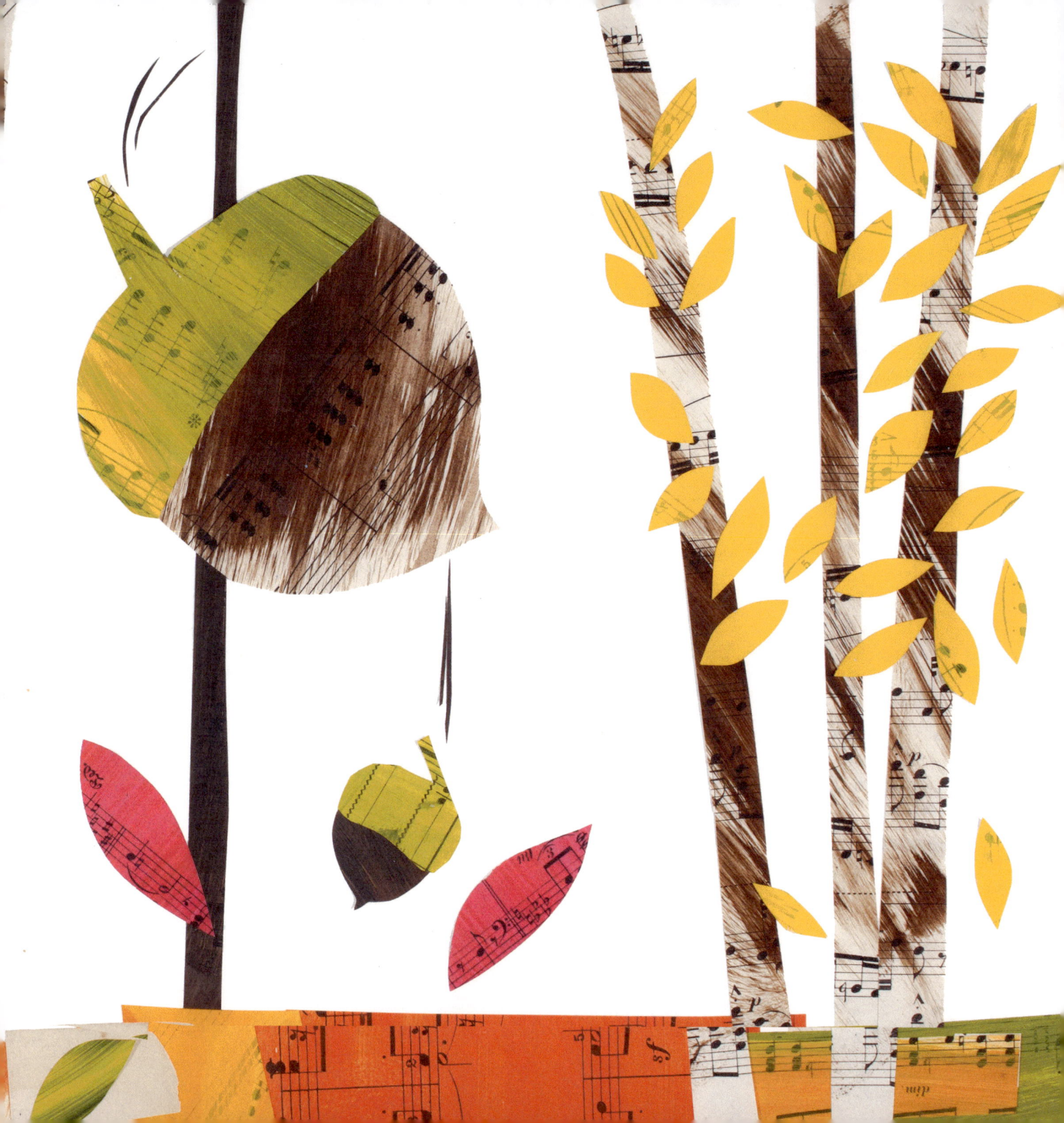

Things I Notice
When I Walk the Dog

Christine Richards

ISBN: 979-8-9857121-0-0

©2022 / Waystation Whistle LLC

Waystation Whistle
PO Box 5290
Portland, ME 04101

Collage illustrations by Christine Richards

All rights reserved. No portion of this book may be used or reproduced in any manner without written permission except for brief quotations in articles or reviews.

Things I Notice When I Walk the Dog

Christine Richards

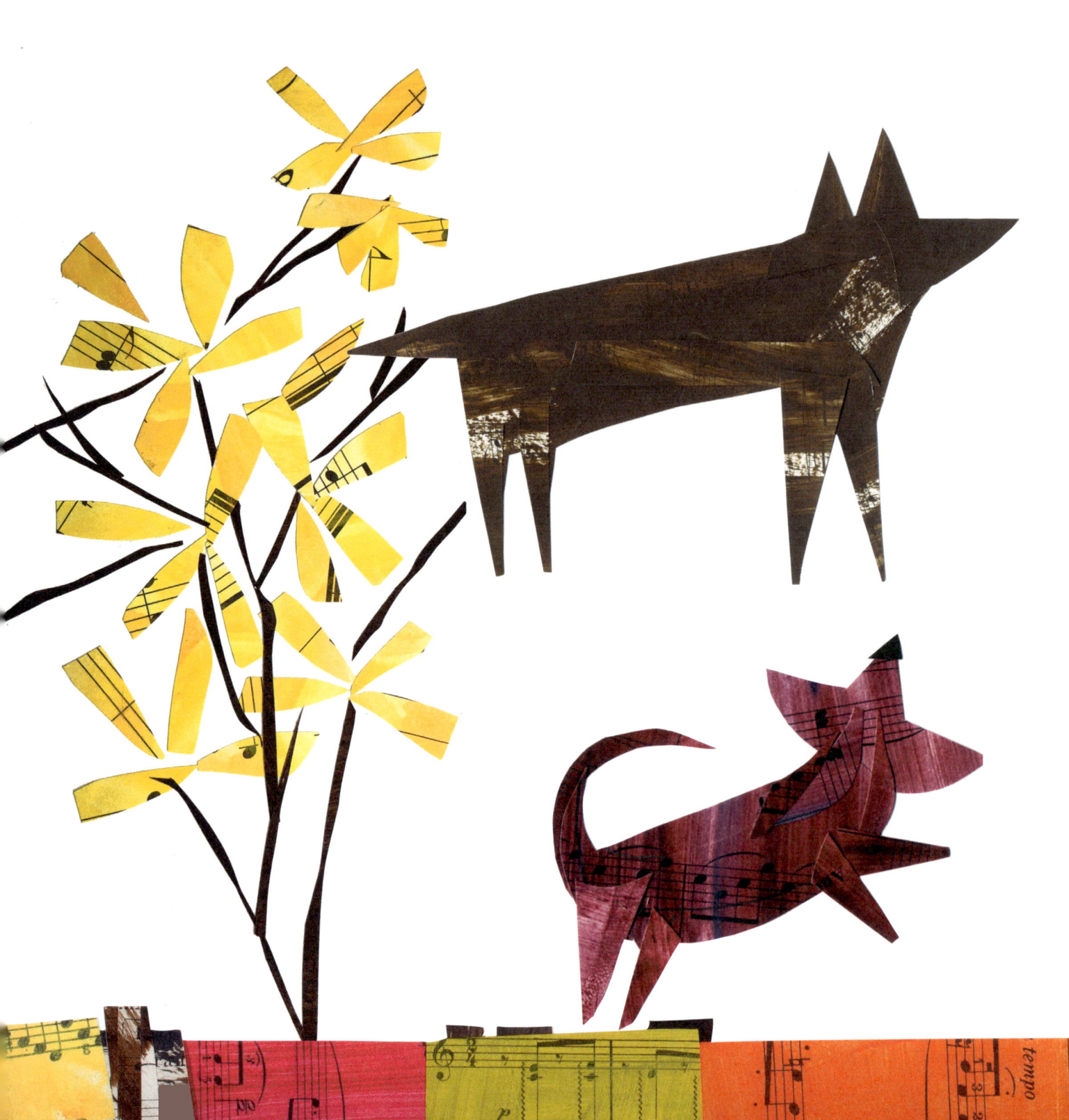

Agatha is a droopy-eyed, long-eared, short-legged, scent-sniffing basset hound.

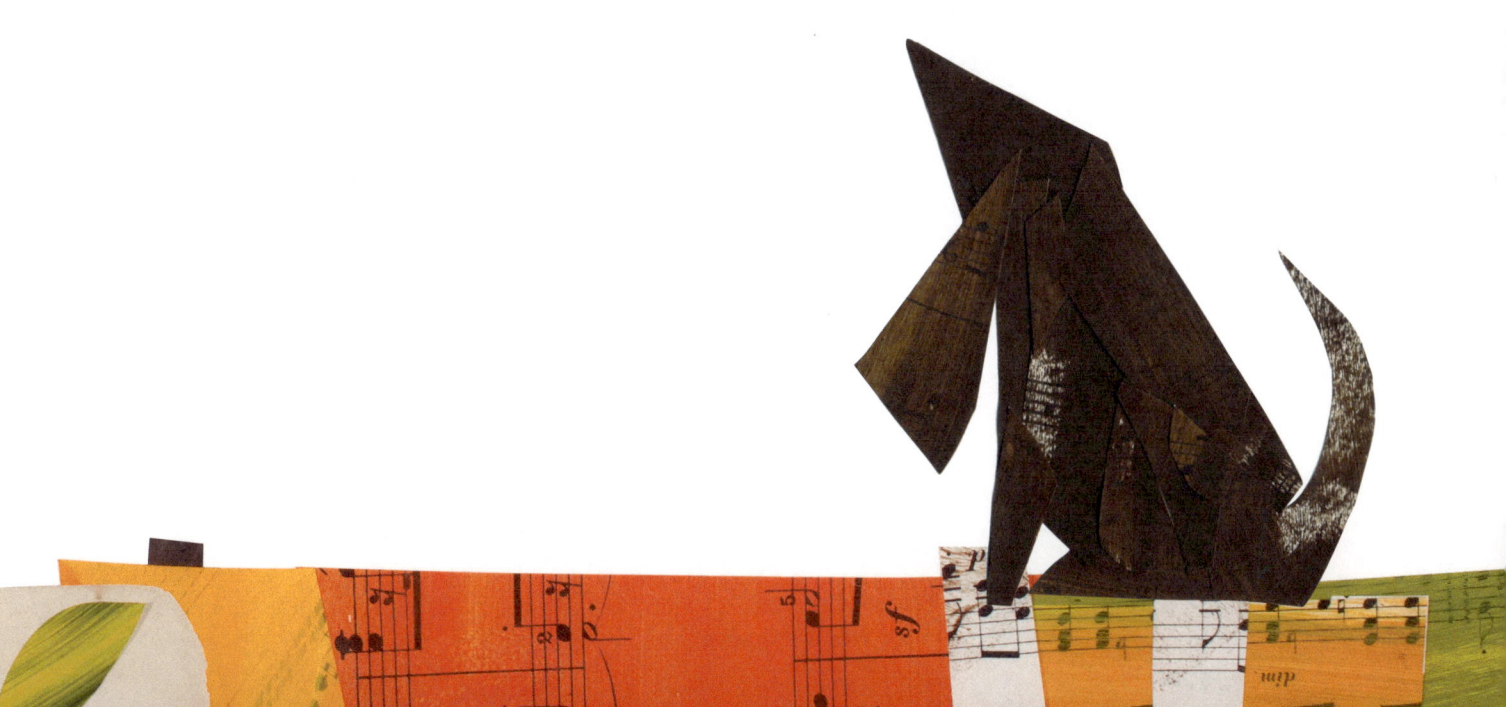

Agatha and I go for a walk every day.

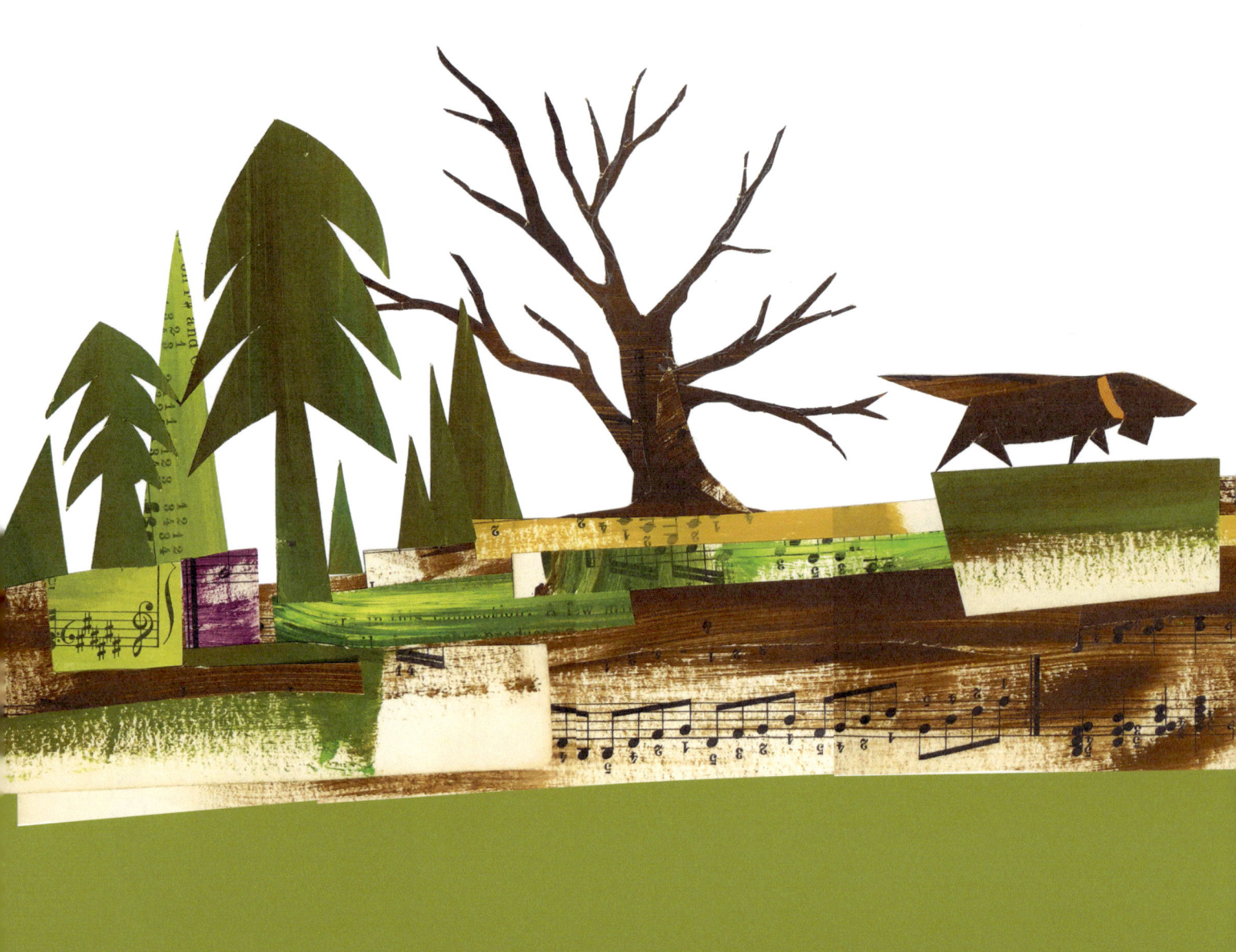

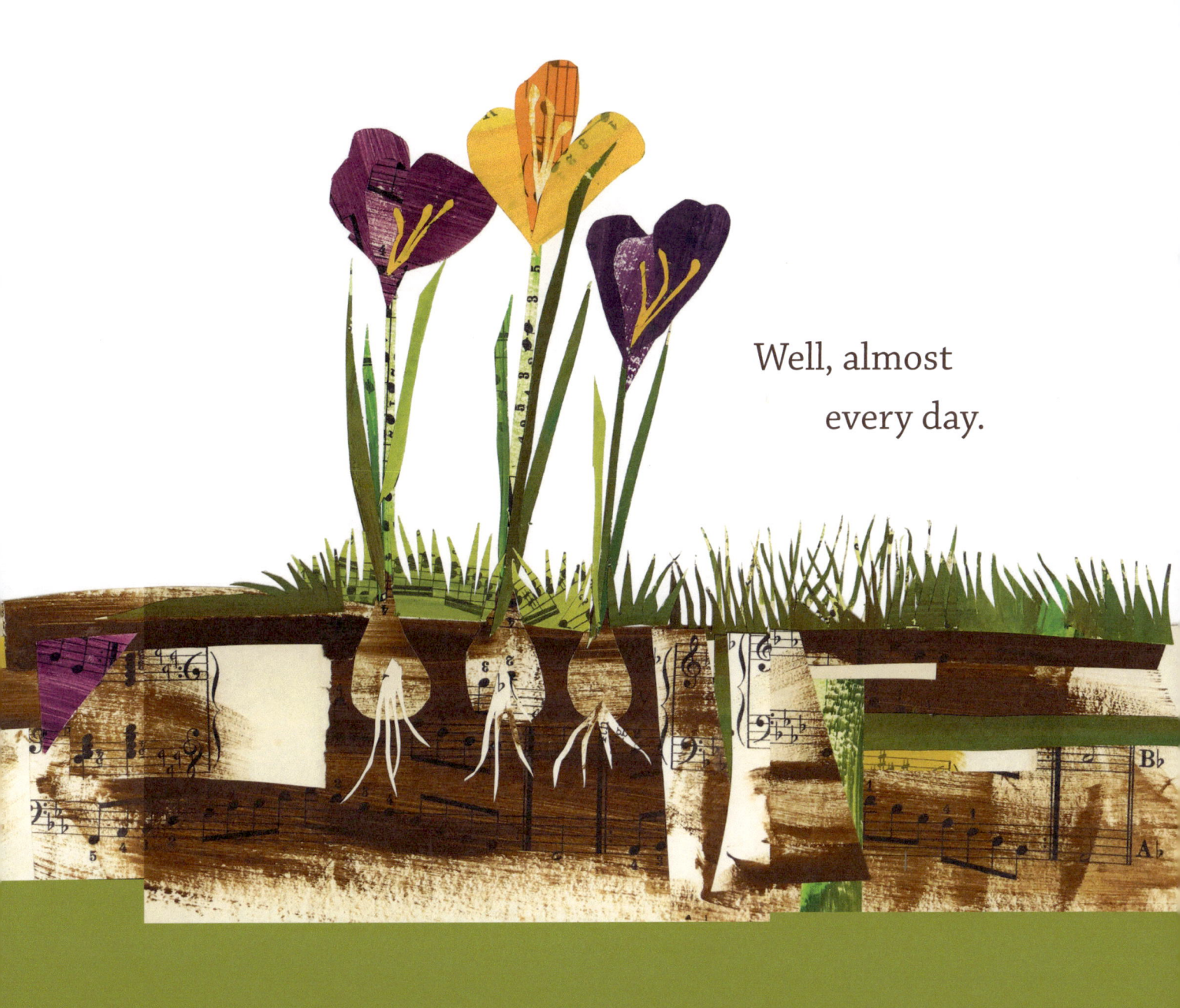

Well, almost every day.

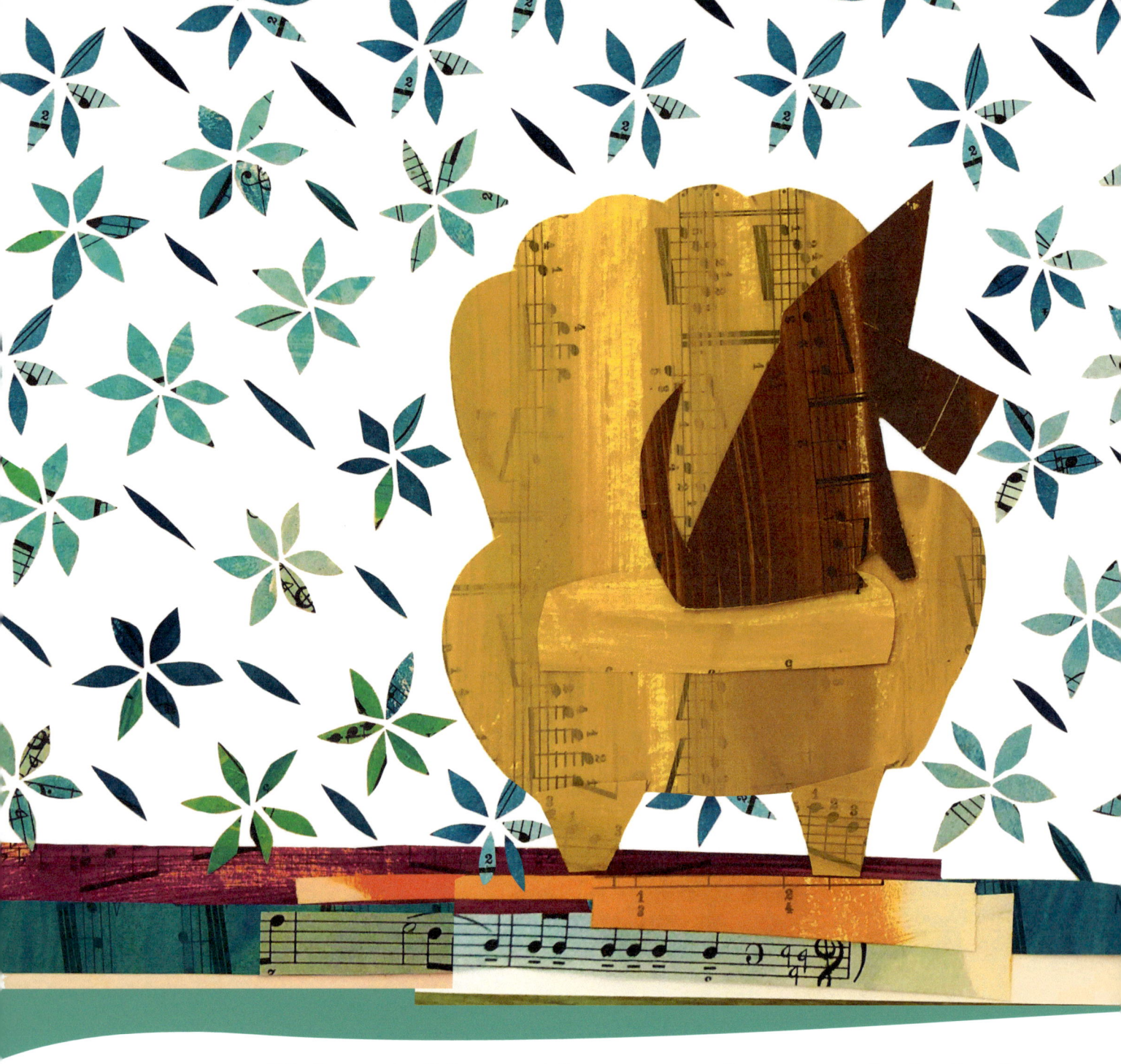

If the rain blows sideways or the snow drifts high

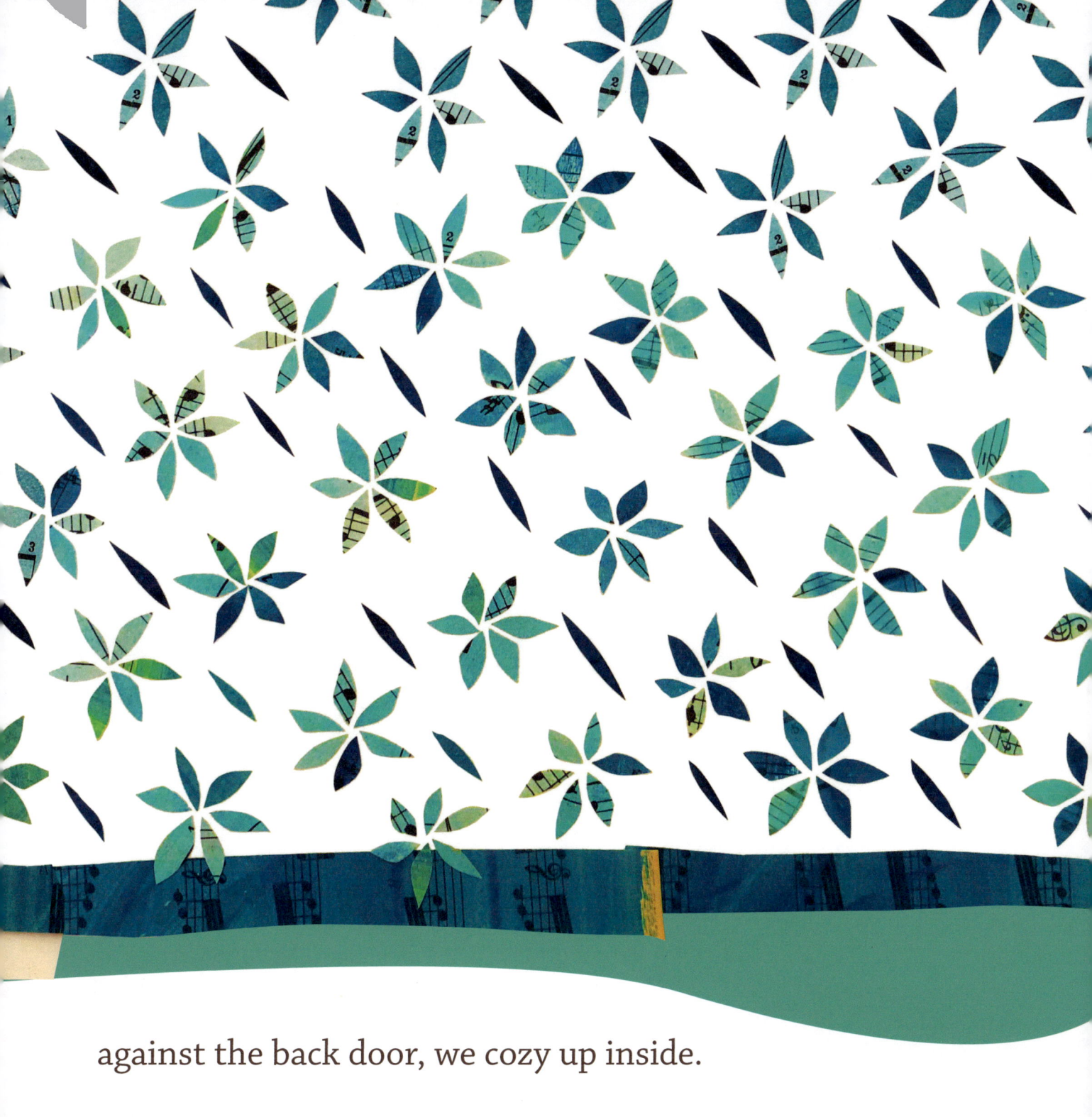

against the back door, we cozy up inside.

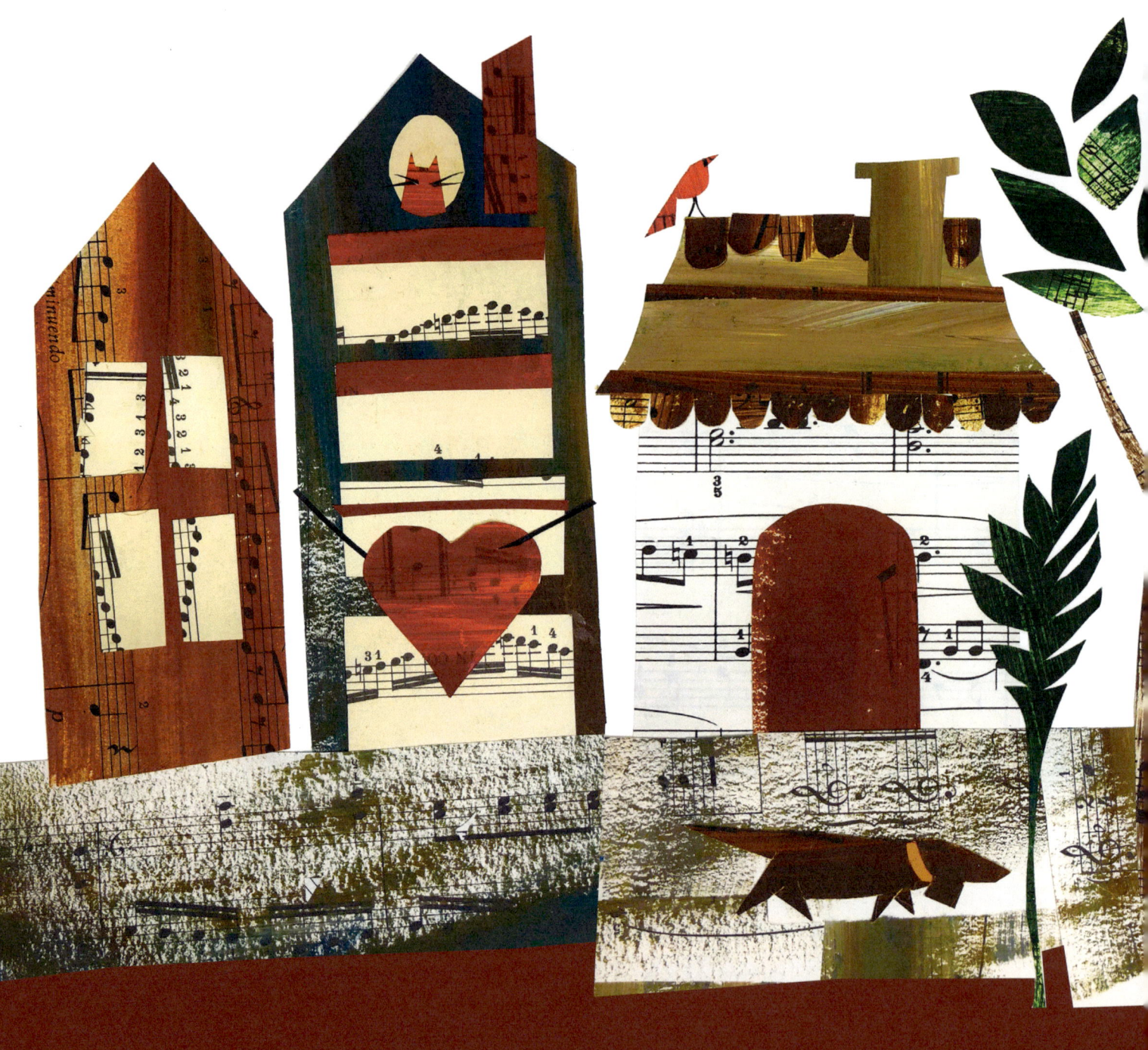

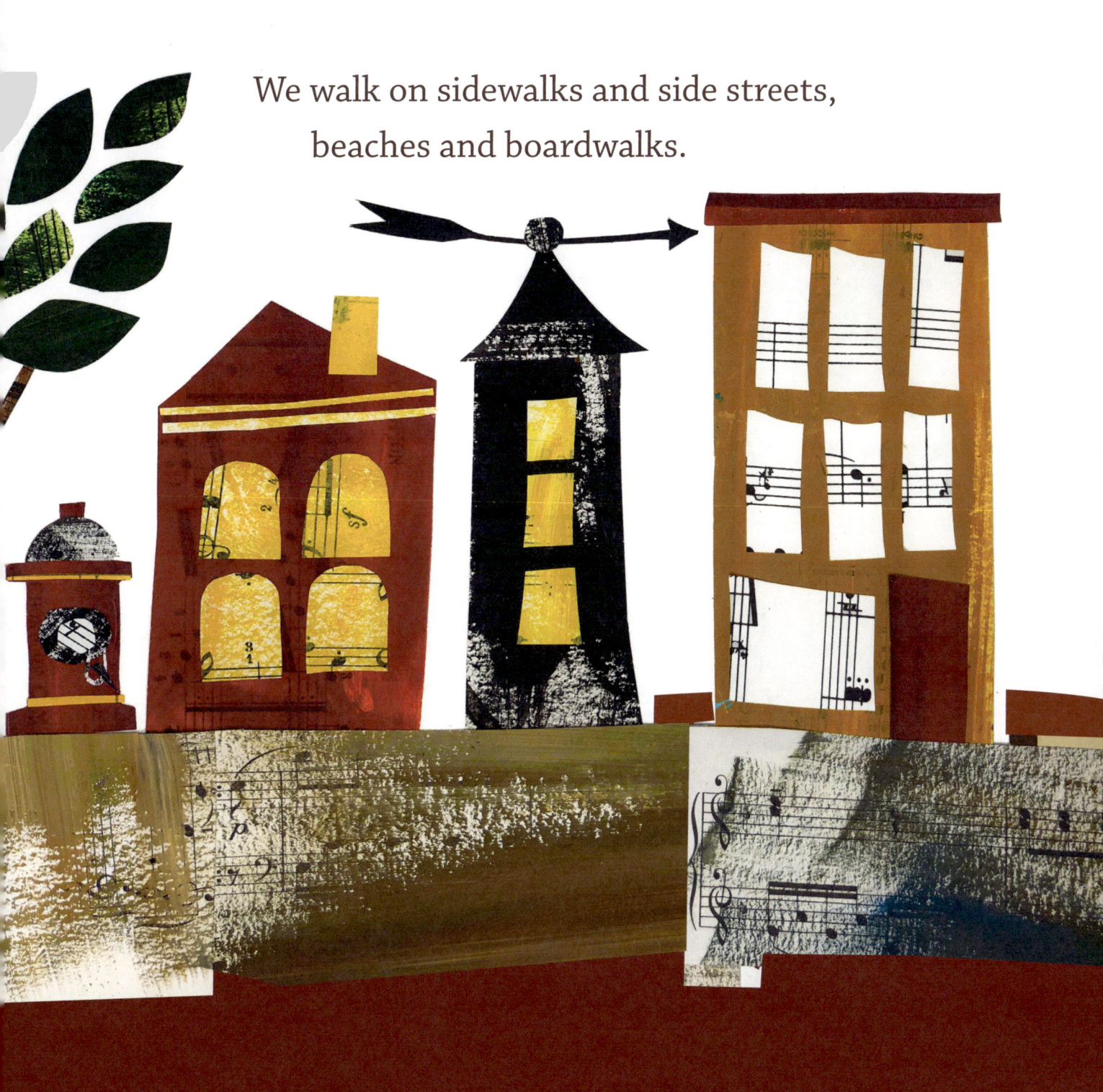
We walk on sidewalks and side streets, beaches and boardwalks.

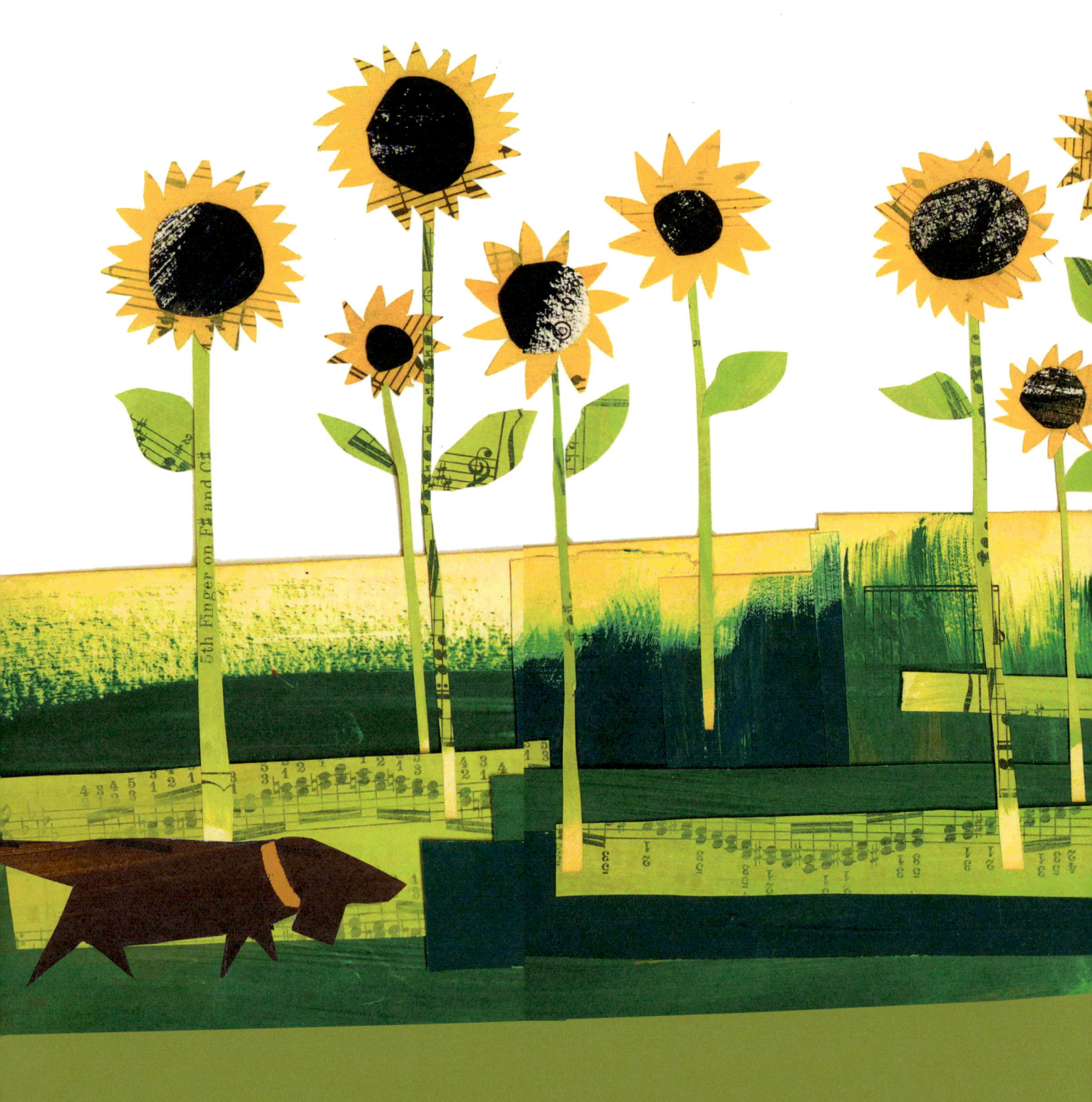

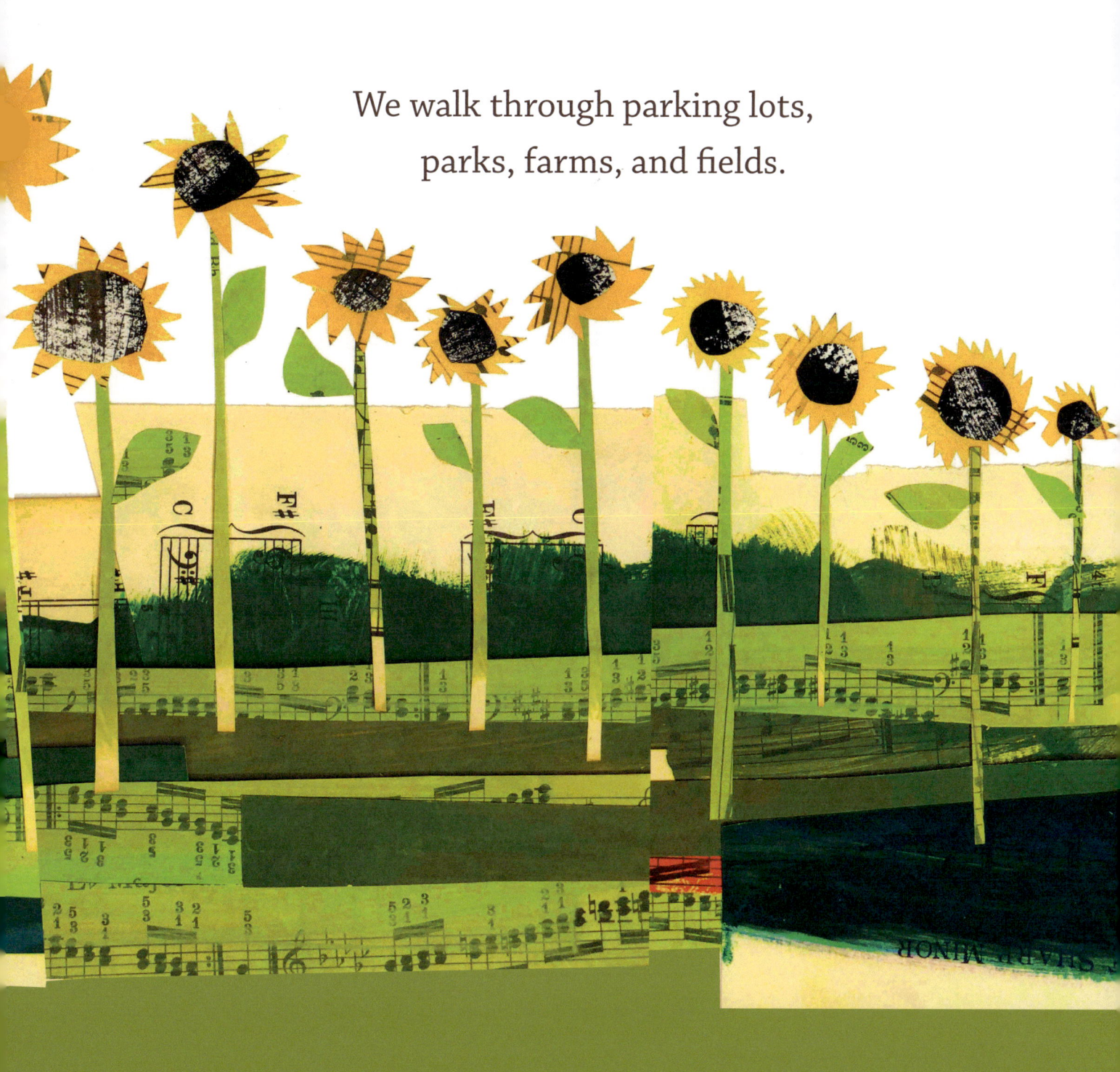

We walk through parking lots,
parks, farms, and fields.

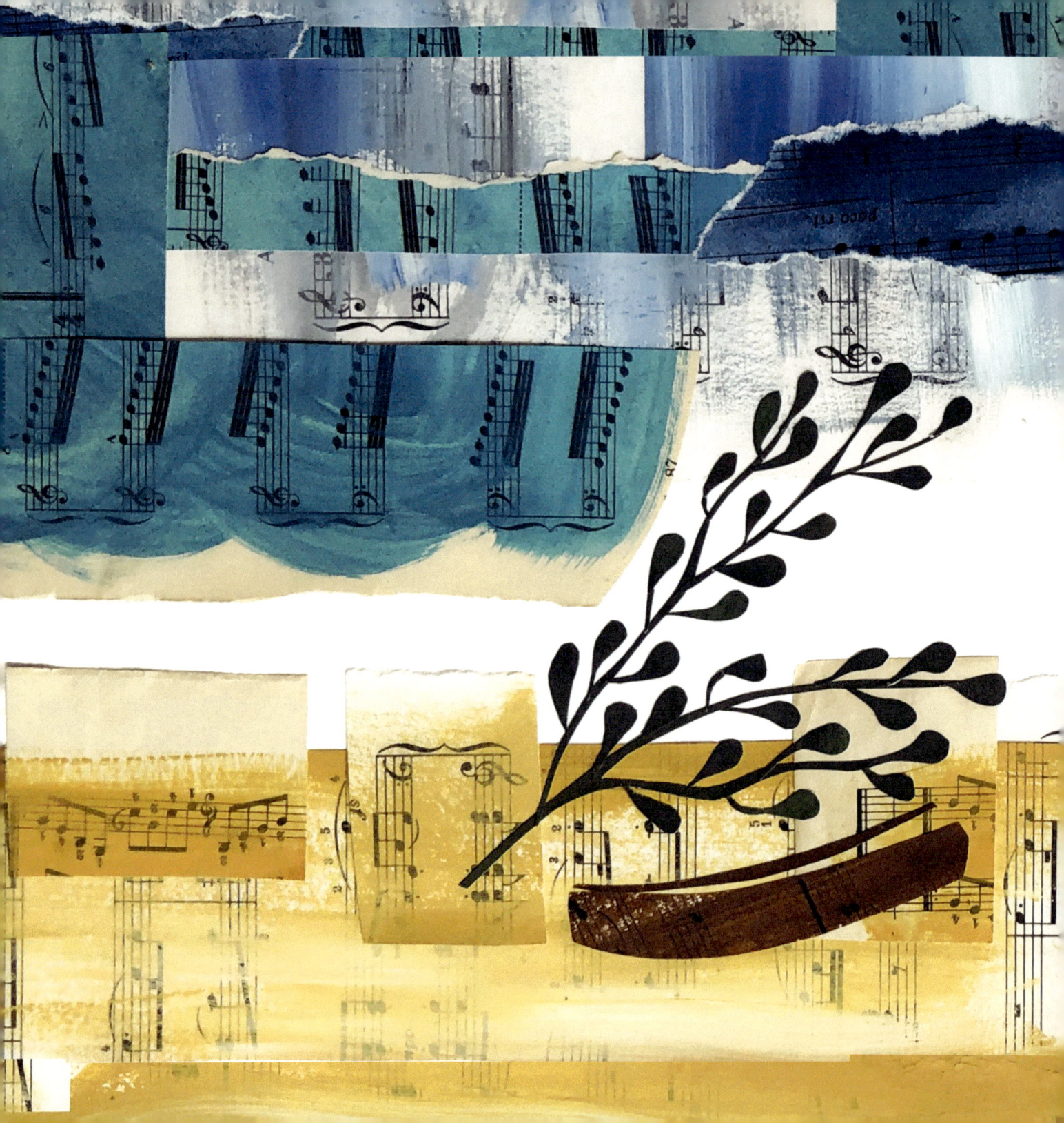

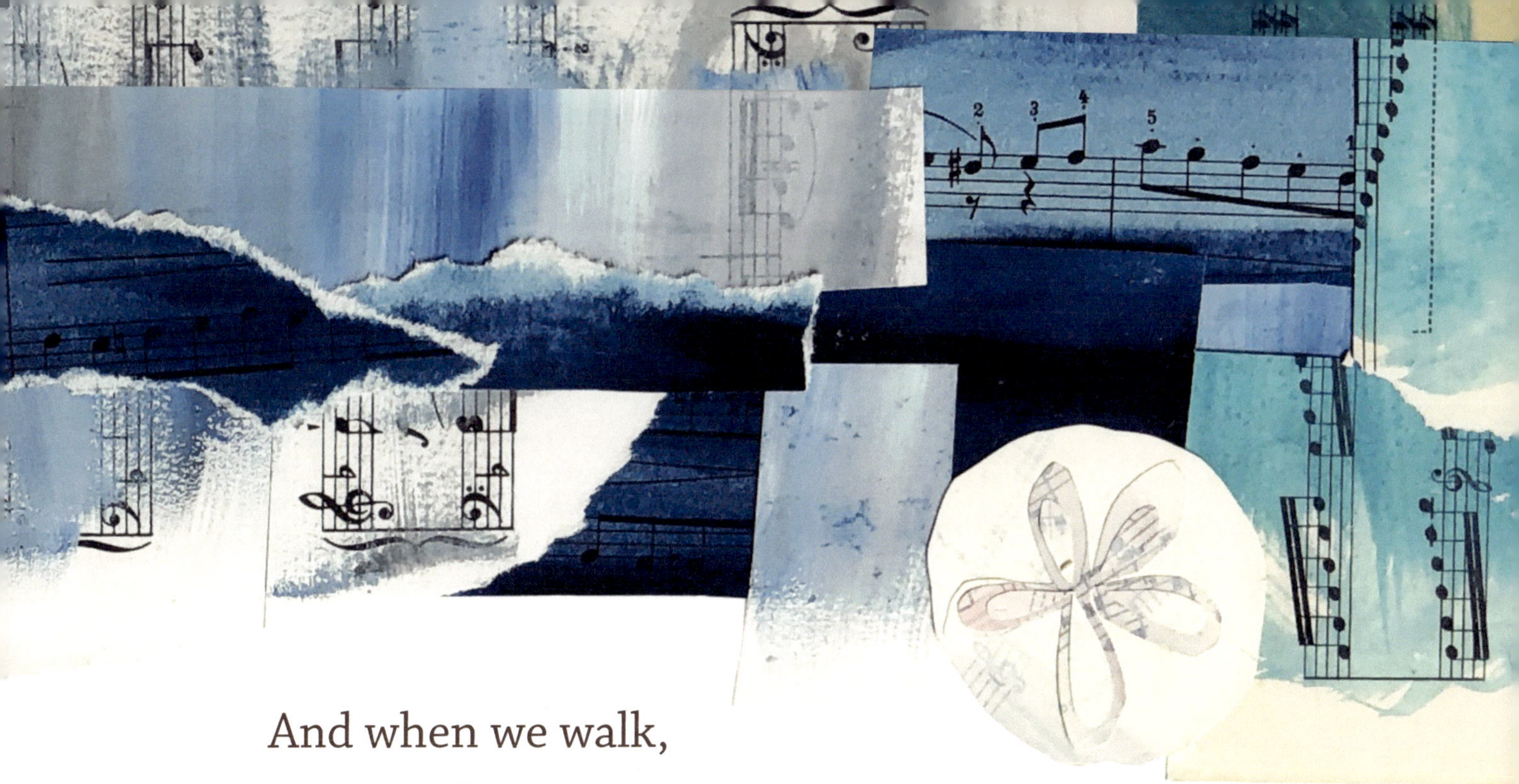

And when we walk,
   Agatha likes to sniff.
      And stop.

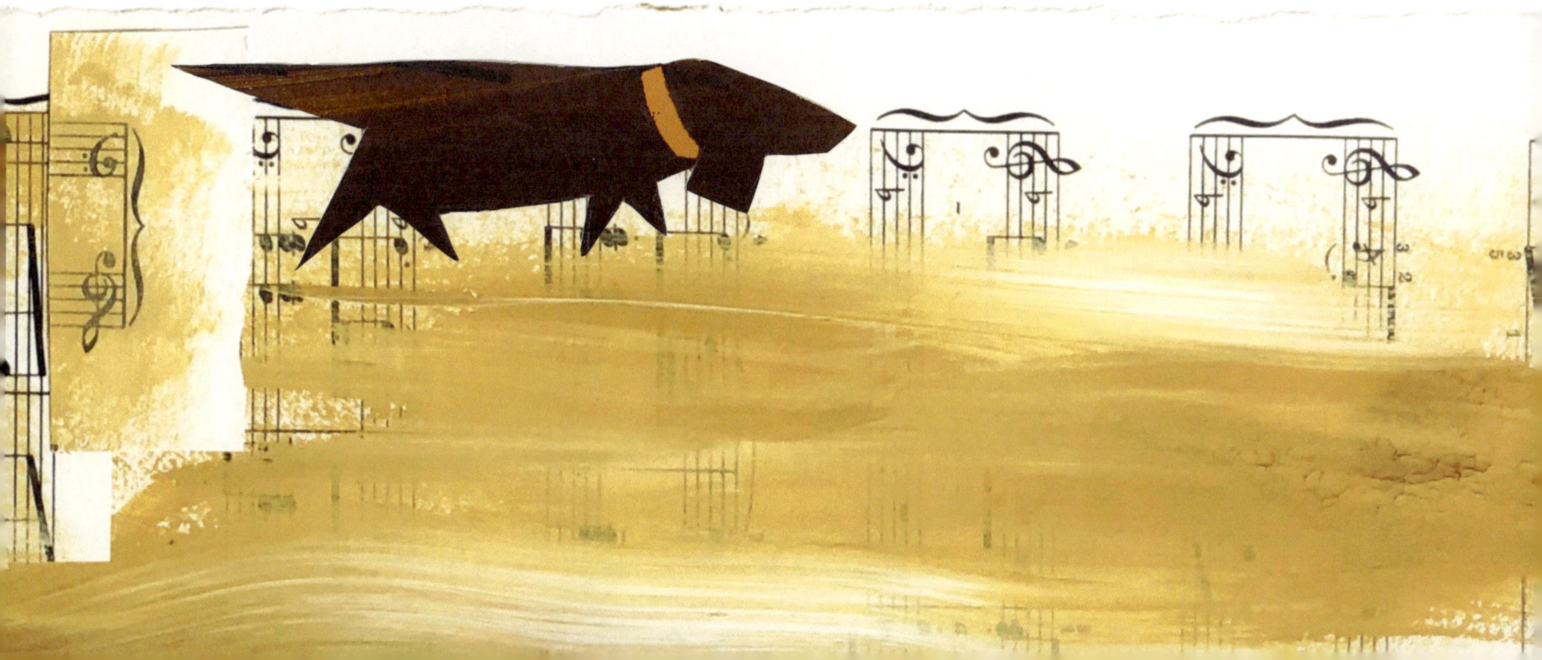

And sniff and stop again.

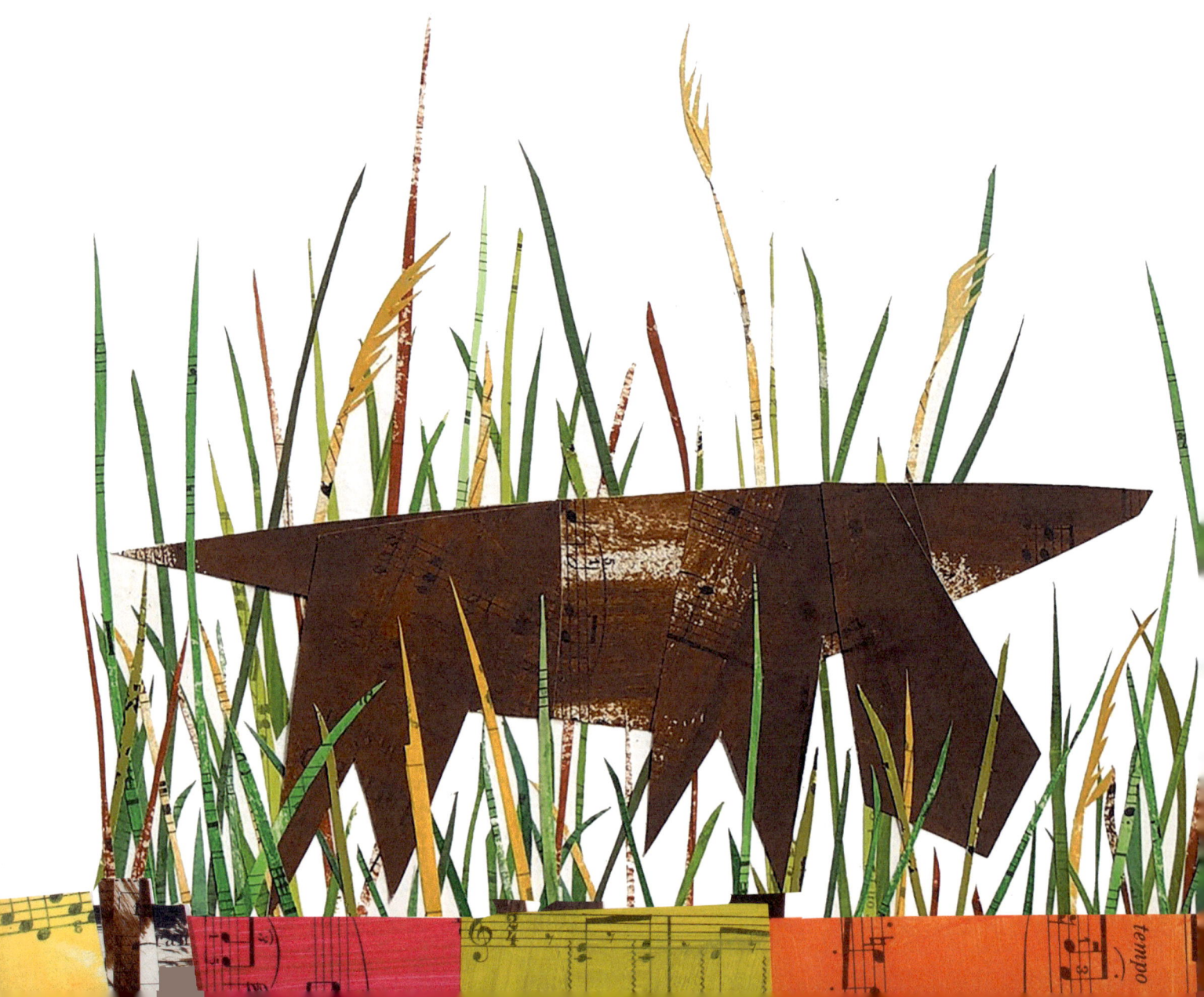

She sniffs at signposts and fence posts, footprints and paw prints, other people, and other dogs.

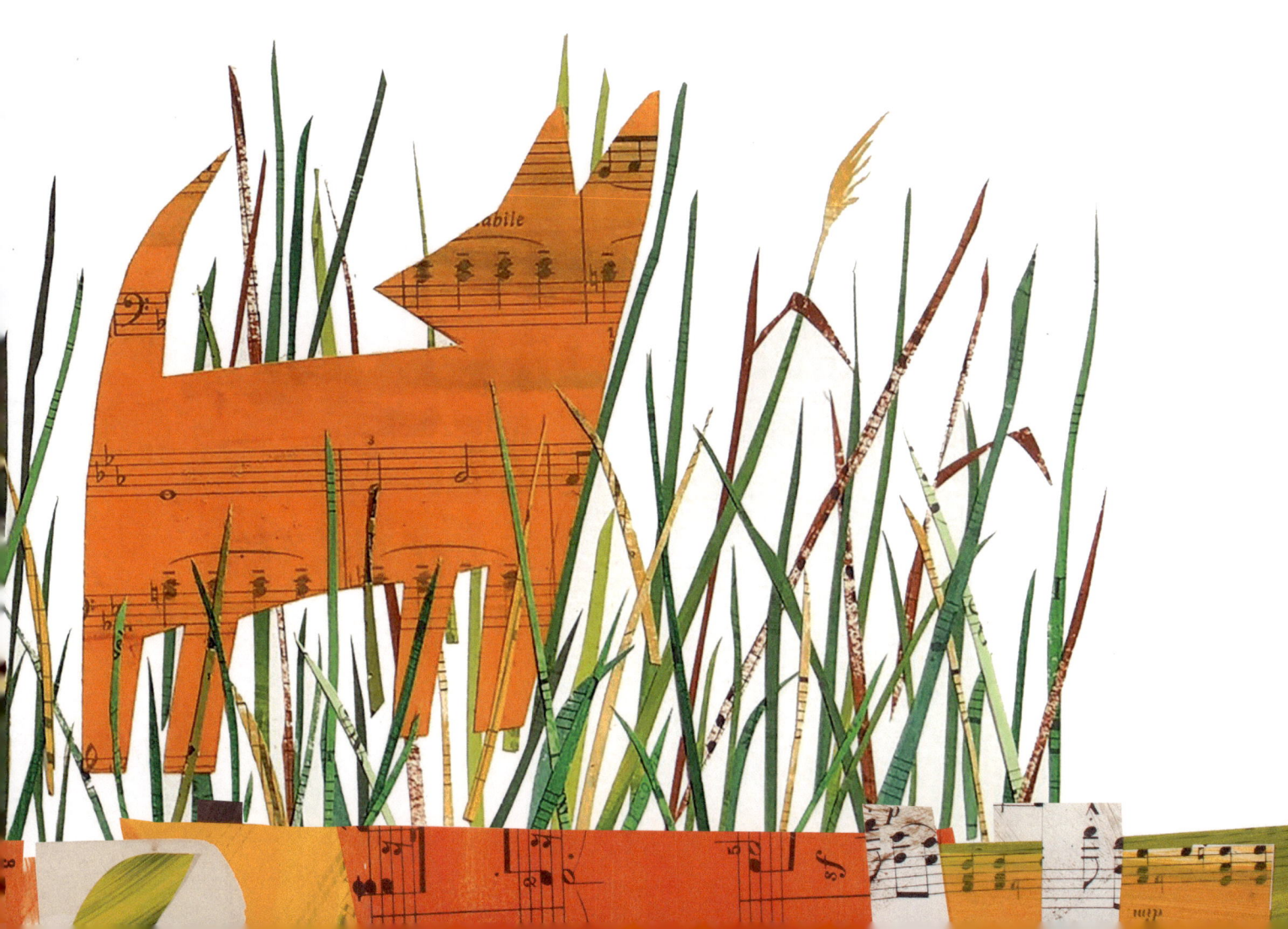

And while she sniffs, I wait.
And while I wait,
I notice things.

I notice morning dew
dampens my sneakers,
pigeons perch on power lines,
cats stop short at the sight of us,
and full moon shadows
follow our lead.

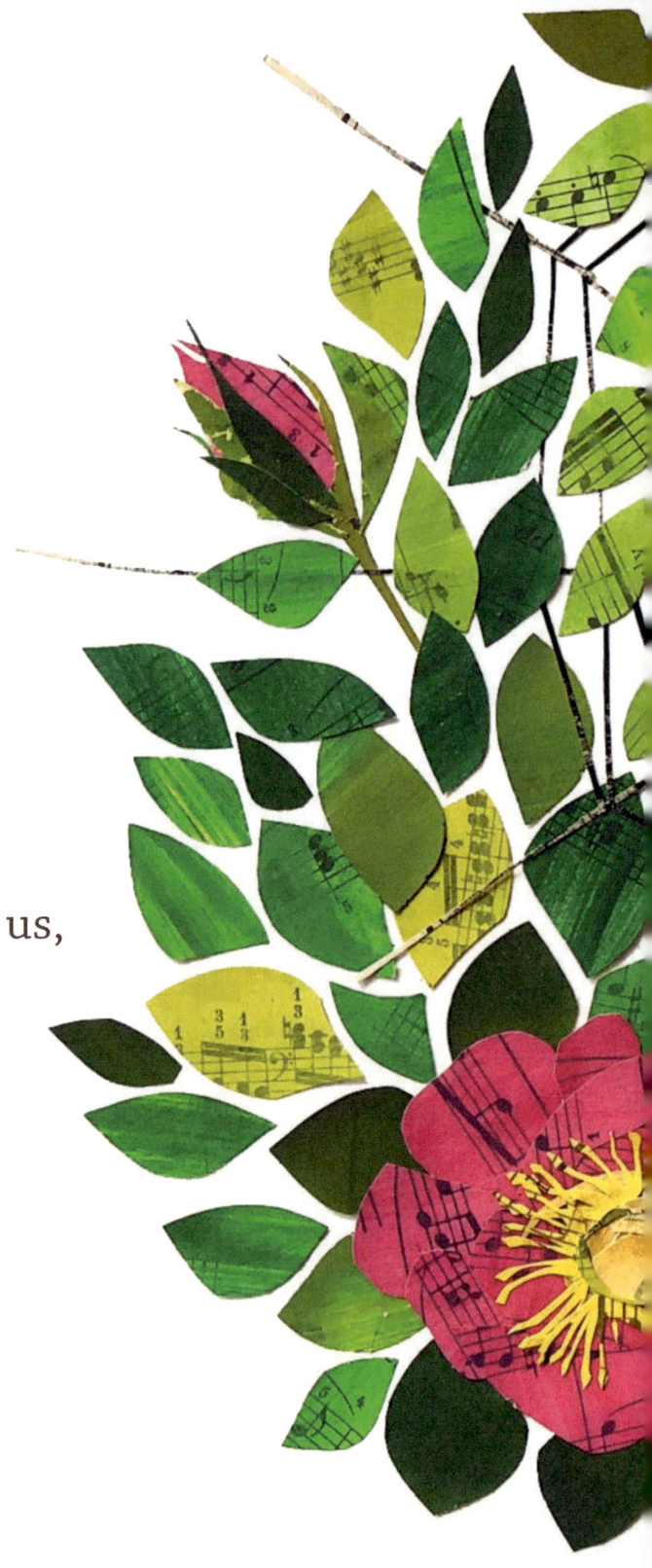

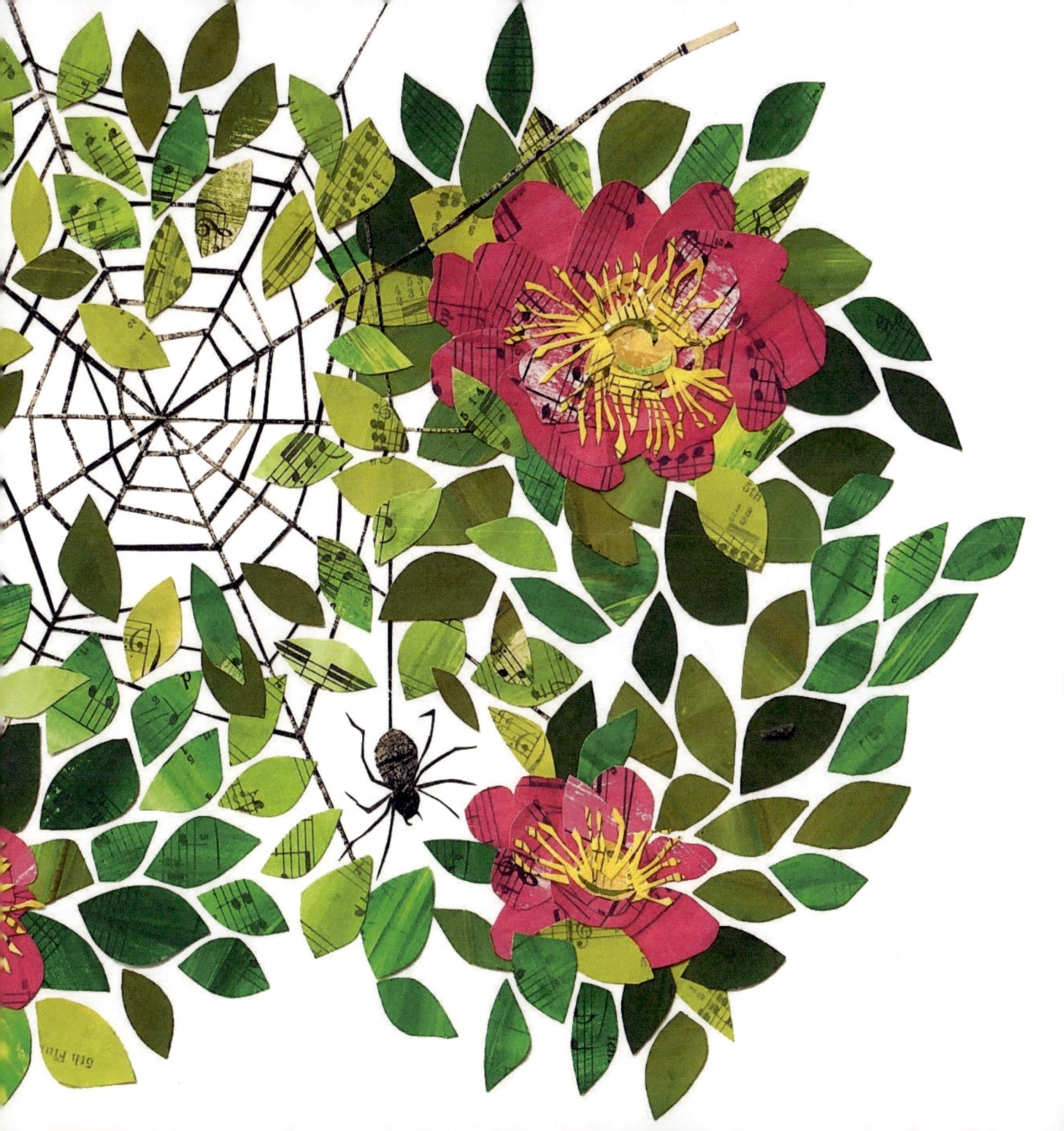

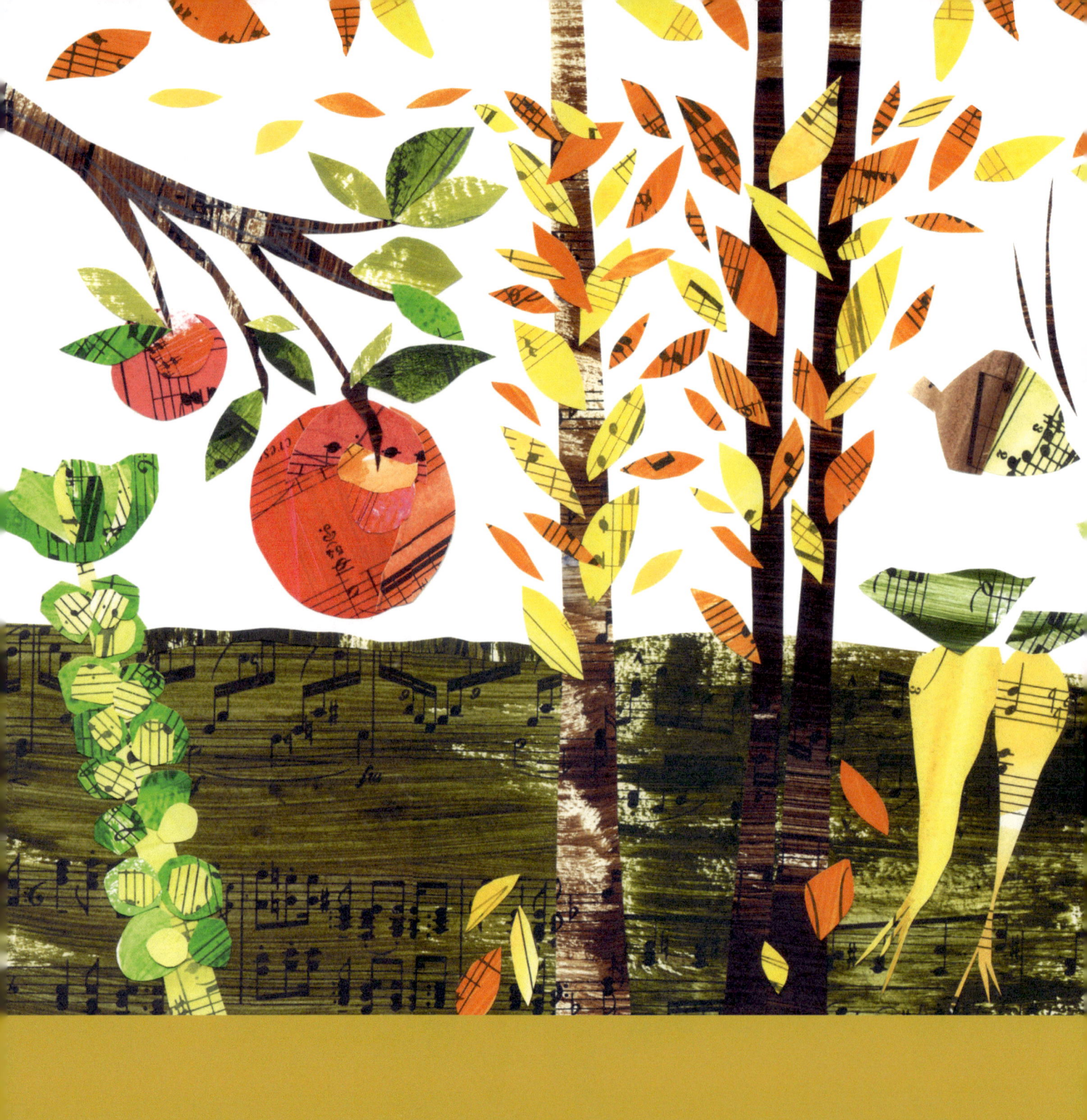

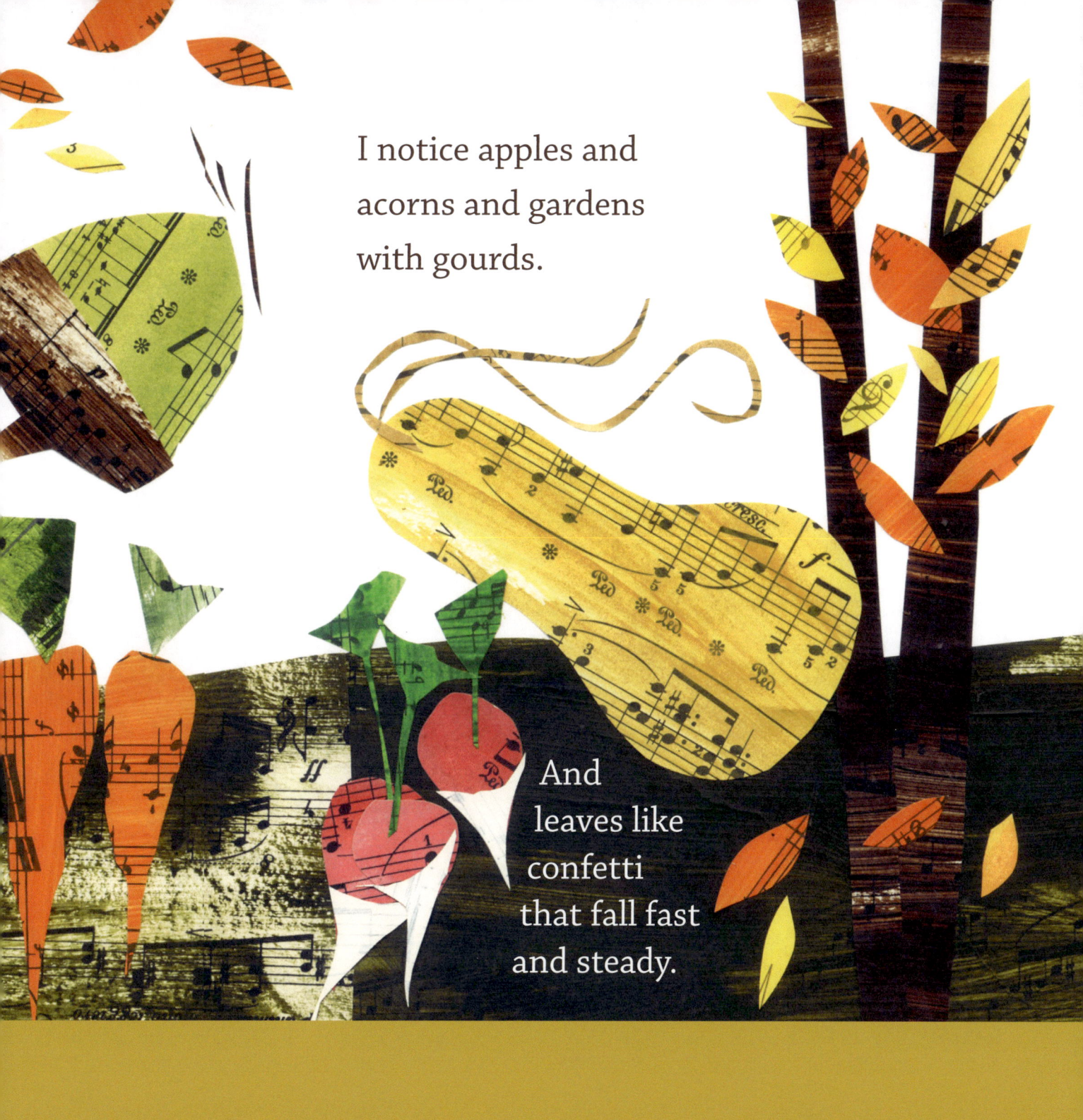

I notice apples and acorns and gardens with gourds.

And leaves like confetti that fall fast and steady.

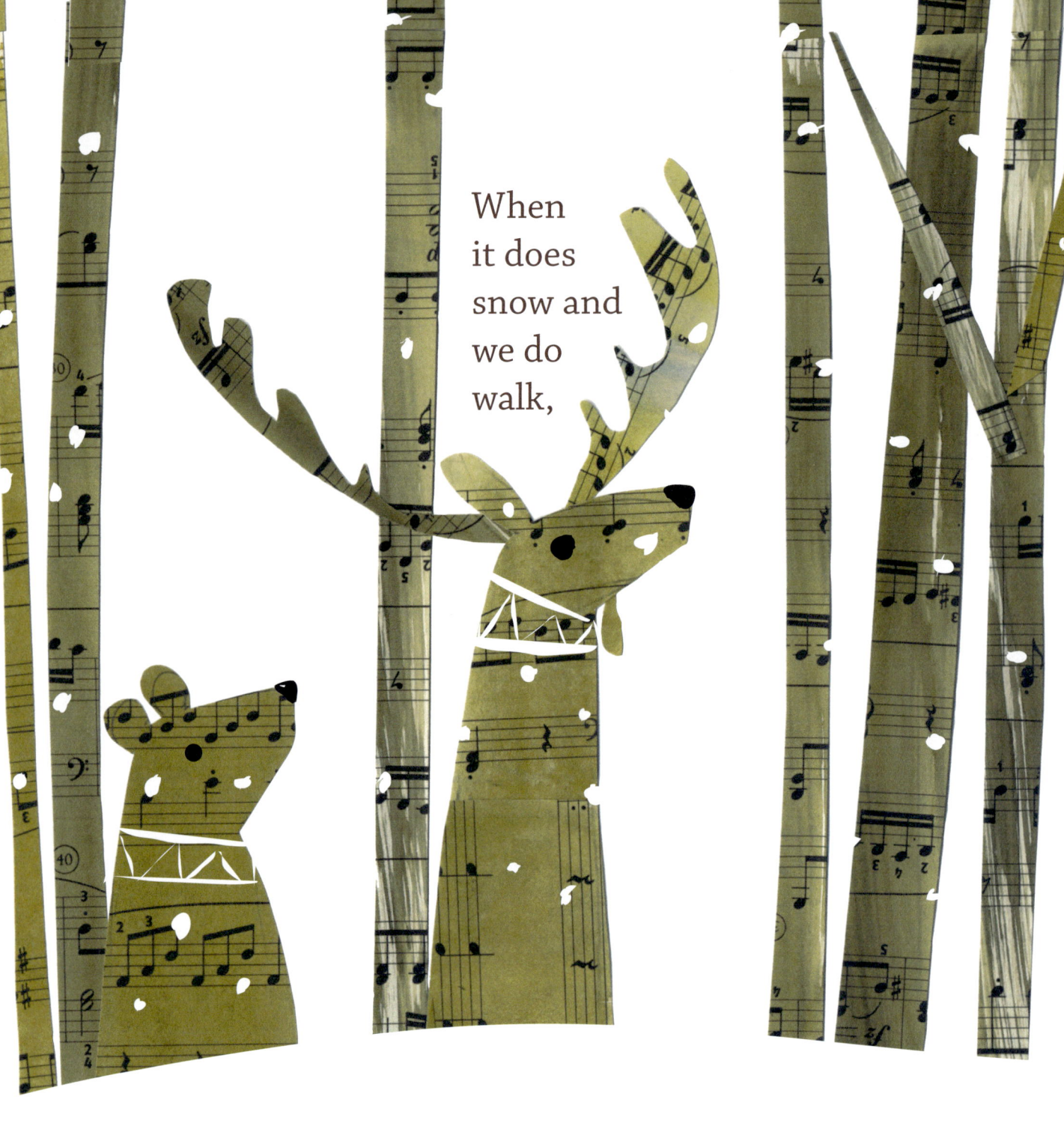

When it does snow and we do walk,

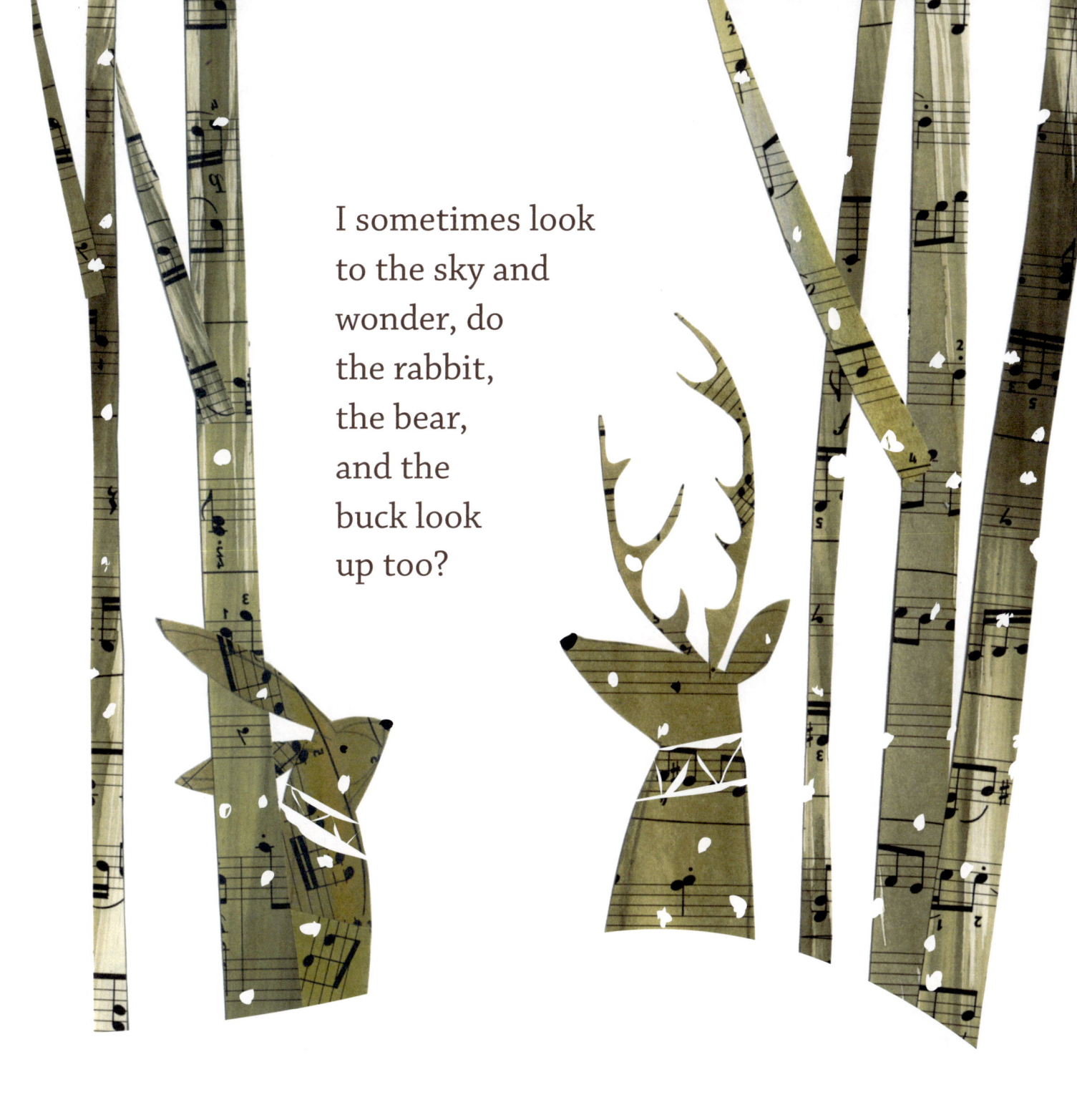

I sometimes look to the sky and wonder, do the rabbit, the bear, and the buck look up too?

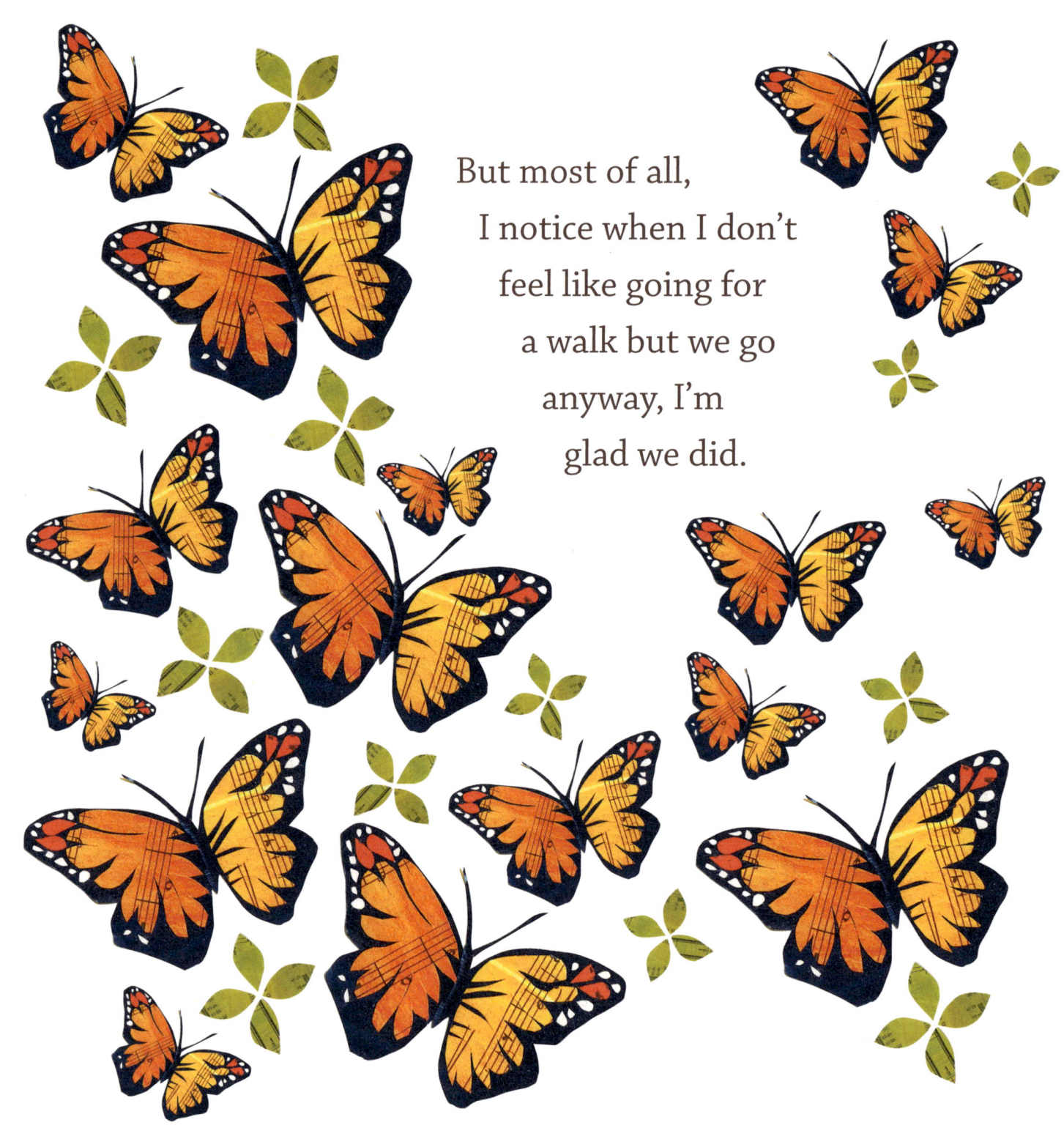

But most of all, I notice when I don't feel like going for a walk but we go anyway, I'm glad we did.

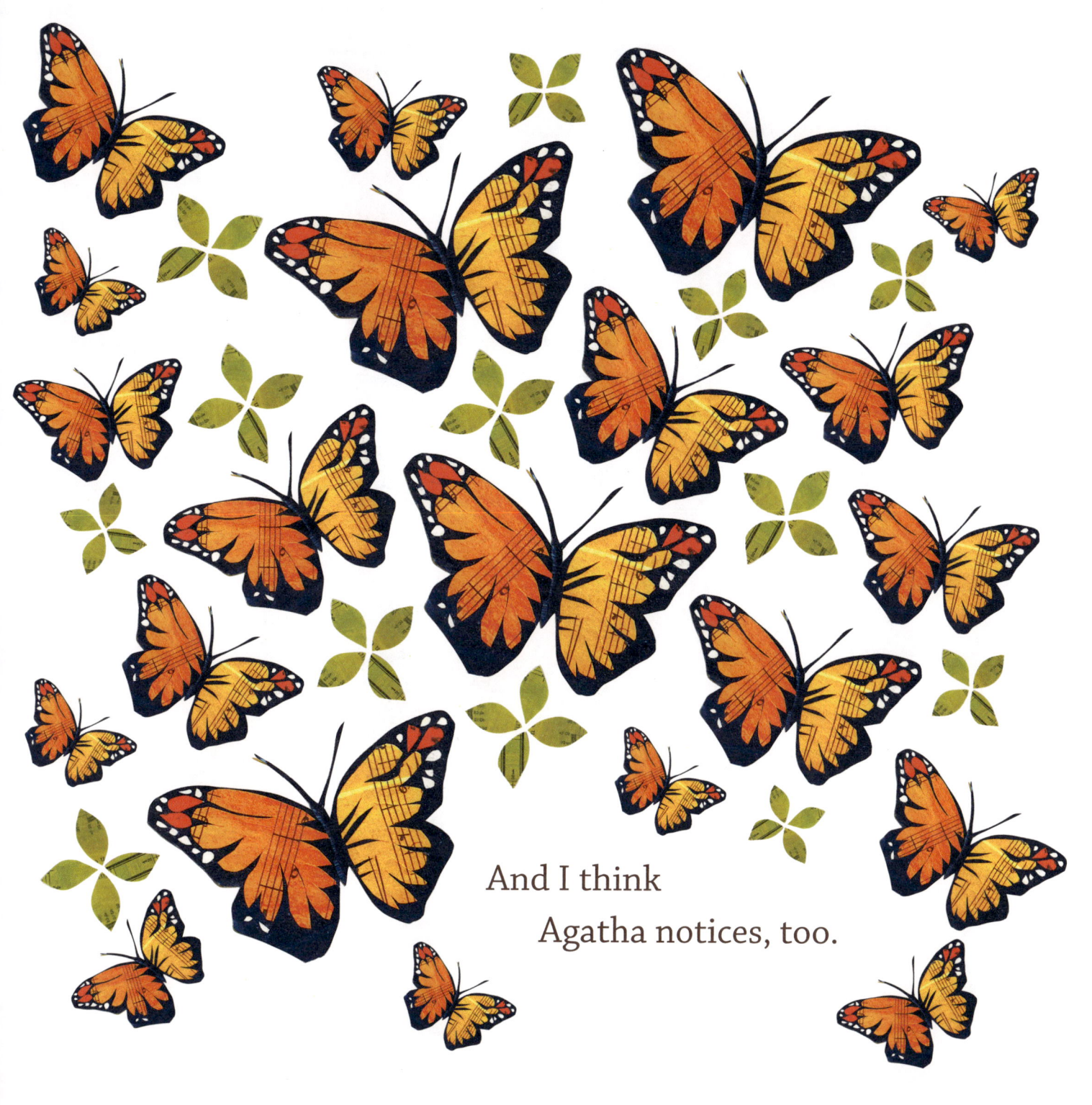

And I think
   Agatha notices, too.

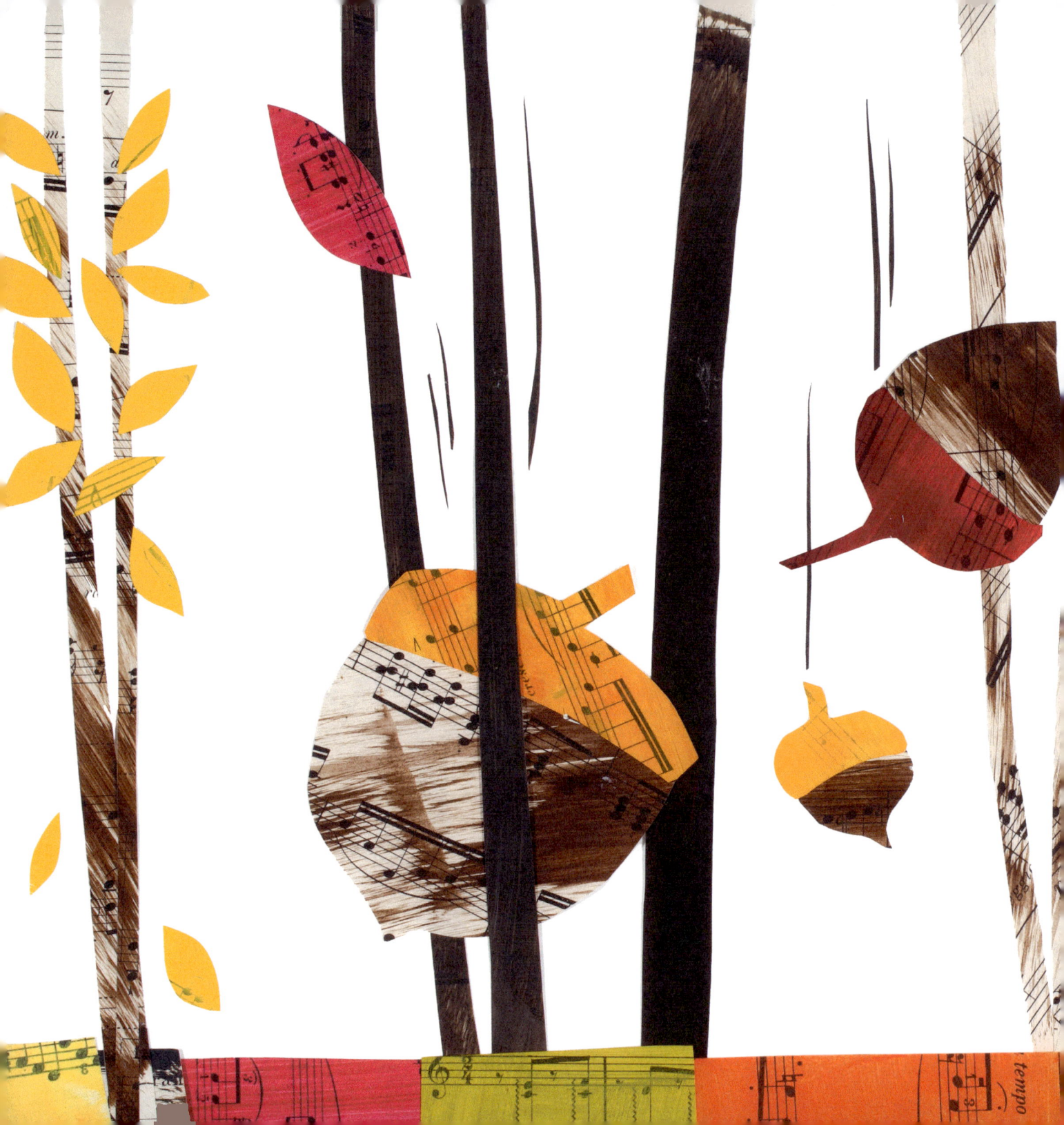

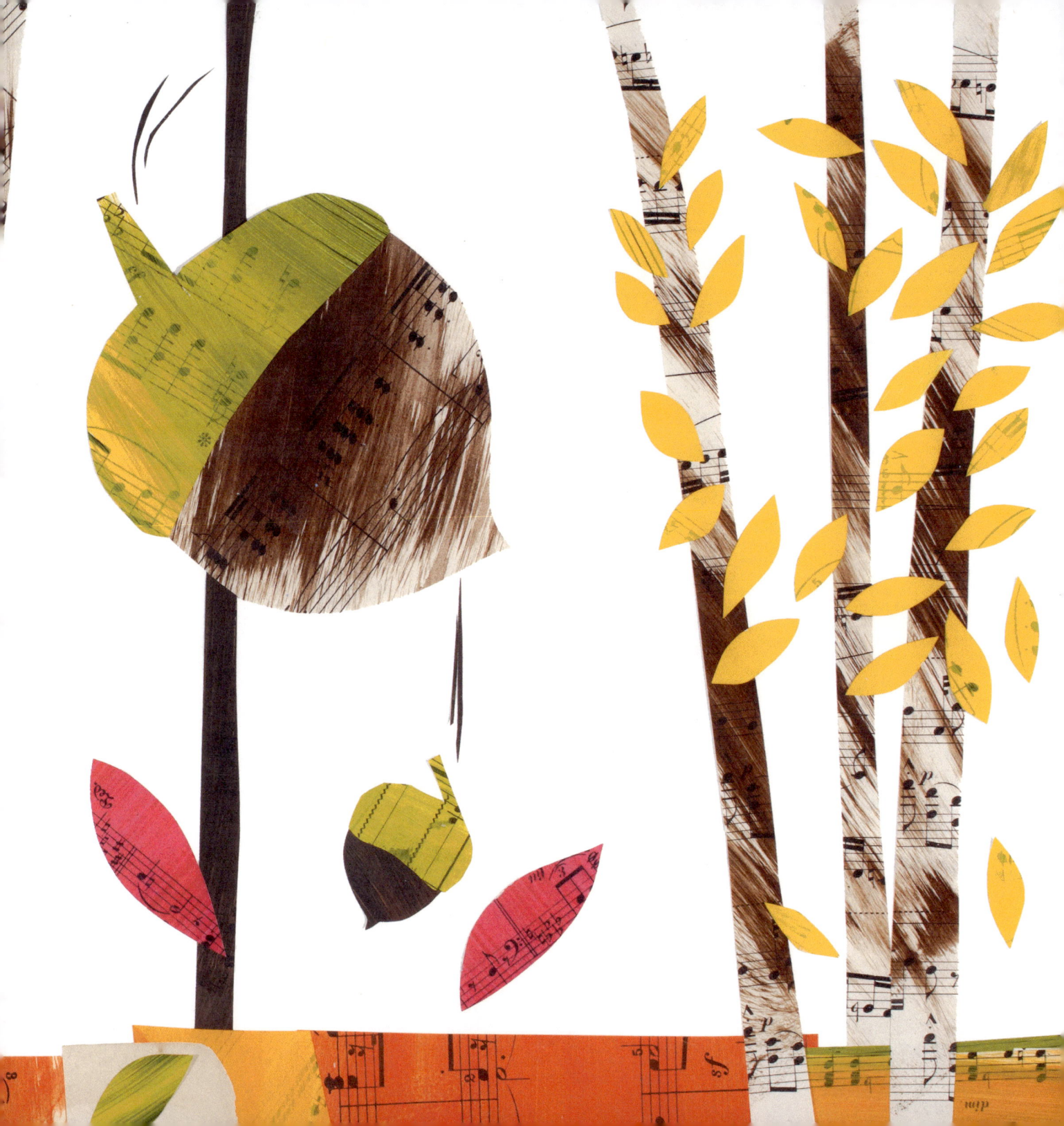

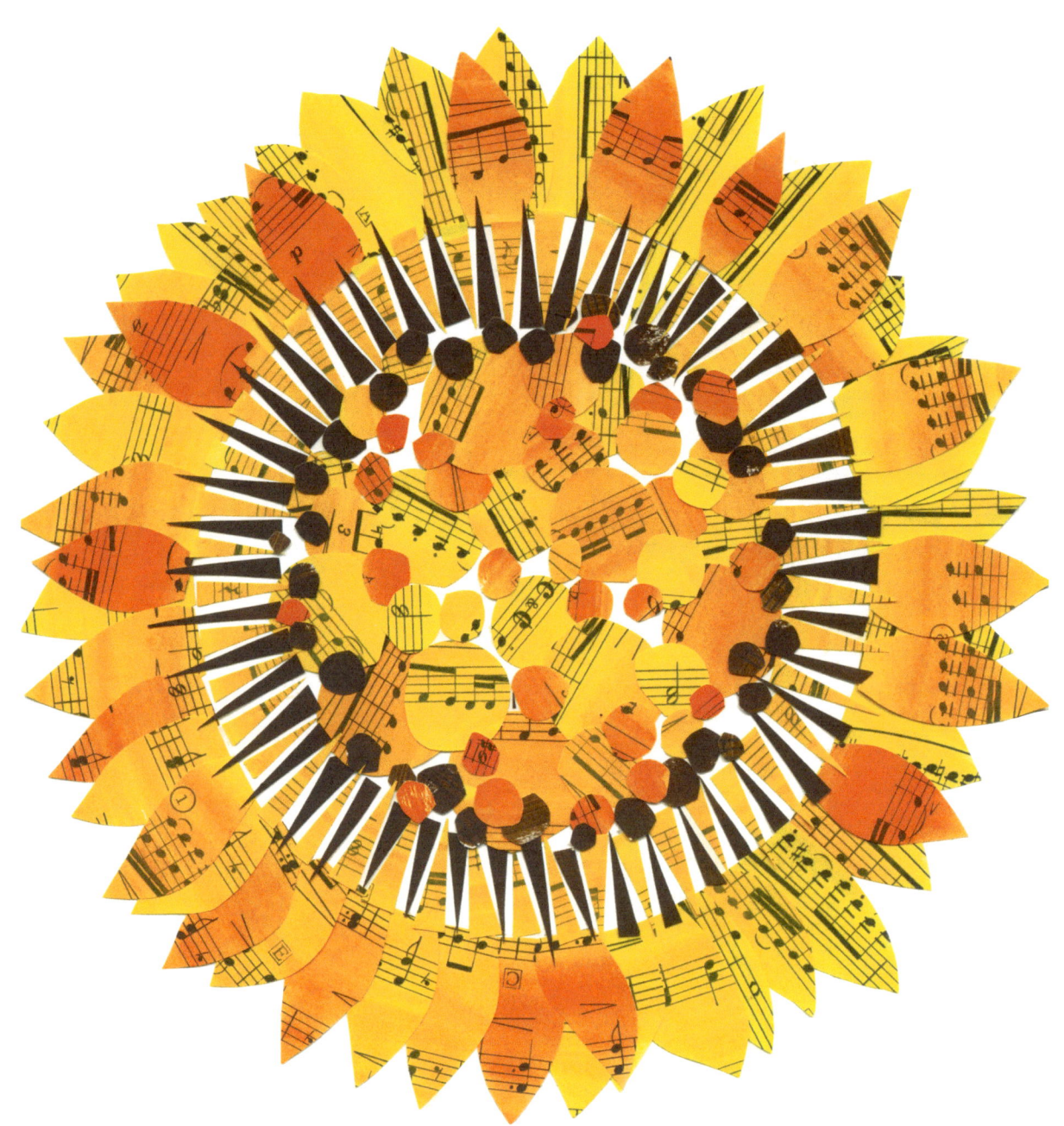

What did you notice?

There are lots of things in the book to notice.
Did you see them all? Here's a list of things to look for:

acorns	sunflowers	cat
spider	weather vane	roses
fire hydrant	forsythia branches	Brussels sprouts
carrots	squash	apples
parsnips	radishes	rabbit
bear	deer	moose
butterflies	seaweed	razor clam
sand dollar	heart	cardinal
crocus flowers	pine trees	chimney

Now it's your turn!
Take a walk and see what there is to notice.

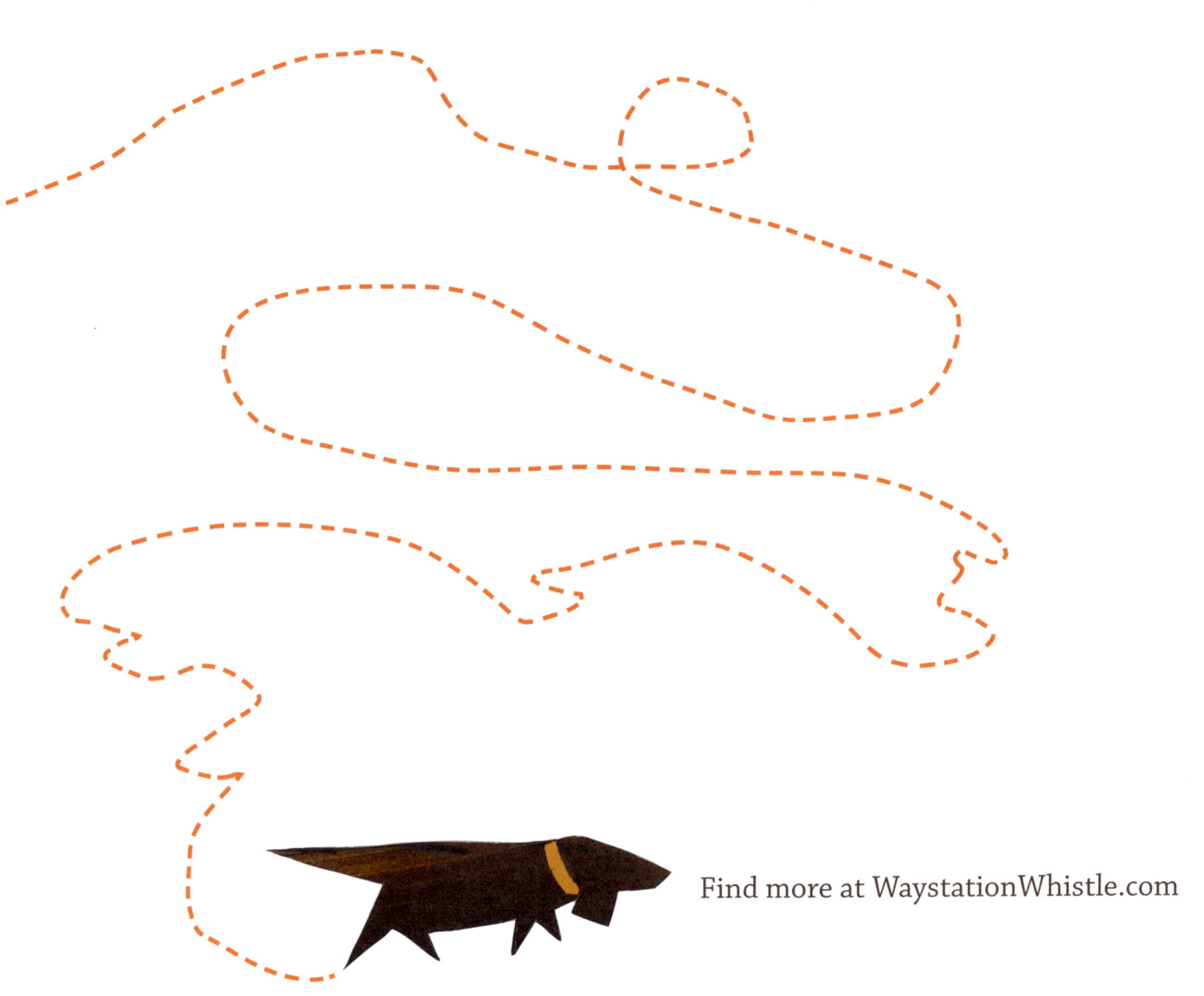

Find more at WaystationWhistle.com

Made in the USA
Columbia, SC
21 December 2024